> To, Mary
> My Dearest old fr
> Enjoy the Read.
>   Best Wishes
>   S. Jones 21.02.2019

My Crazy Cell Mate

Susan Jones

INTRODUCTION

This is a true story about my journey with a meningioma Brain Tumour. It is written with all I can remember and my diary of events, which I used to charter my recovery as my short term memory was confused and non-existent.

My Family, Friends, Neighbours, and those who knew me well, have filled in some of the gaps with what actually happened. They have enabled me to put this all together. If I repeat myself, which is quite often it is part of my condition, it is not done intentionally. It is the way I have taught myself to retain information; anything else is unfortunately lost.

I hope anyone else out there going through a similar journey finds inspiration and comfort that we are not going mad and there is a life to have that's worth living.

ABOUT ME

I am a 58 year old Yorkshire lass, a single mum with one daughter.

I wanted to write my story to help others going through a similar experience and to give people hope about this life changing disease.

I want to raise money for Brain Tumour Research to repay the wonderful NHS who without their excellent care I would not be here today and to improve treatment for future patients.

It is my way of giving something back to say Thank you for giving me a second chance, without the skills, dedication and commitment of the neurological teams my life would have been so very different.

The proceeds of my book sales are being donated for further research.

CONTENTS

1. BEFORE DIAGNOSIS
2. MY JOURNEY TO RECOVERY
3. COMING HOME
4. REHABILITATION
5. LIFE GOES ON

1.

BEFORE DIAGNOSIS

I guess it all started around the year 2012, that's when everything started to go downhill, my health was deteriorating slowly. I believed my symptoms were because of my age, 52 and overworking and experiencing menopause. I convinced everyone else, or so I thought, as I was known for working very long hours and never taking time off for myself, I even got a certificate once for having more energy than the national grid.

I loved my job: it was my life and my baby. I loved a challenge and wouldn't stop until it was to my satisfaction. I've worked in hospitality for 13 years. I was very driven to make the hotel the best it could be. With my staff to work alongside me, I built up a great team who all worked hard and worked well together. It wasn't all hard work-we had social outings and helped each other when problems arose. I was the manager of the housekeeping team and Duty manager most weekends, it was a very hard and physical job, not many people could stick it for long as it was back-breaking and fast-paced and also very target driven. I was hands on and always ready to learn something new.

I started to feel very tired all the time and couldn't seem to get enough sleep no matter what time I went to bed. I told everyone I met how tired I was, but still I carried on until eventually I couldn't do my job anymore. I was forever in trouble getting sent to performance reviews, questioned all the time, I couldn't fathom what I was doing wrong, I thought they were picking on me because they wanted to put someone else in my position so I asked if I could move down to a less pressurized post as I was very tired and upset and I didn't want to be sacked. I've been a single parent for a long time, had hard times and lots of battles to keep my home and a roof over our heads, the last thing I wanted was to be homeless at my age. The management agreed and I was given the position of housekeeping supervisor. I did this for a year according to my contract, but I have no recollection of doing this: my memory was fading.

I was, once again, getting sent for performance reviews because I still was not fulfilling my duties. I just couldn't understand what the problems were; I thought my work was ok. I got it into my head that they wanted me out but I wouldn't give in, I couldn't.

After another review I once again asked if I could move to another position in the hotel where there was no responsibility as I just could not cope. They thought about it and decided I could have a job in the restaurant as a breakfast team member. I started in August 2013 and by May 2014 I was in trouble, I was in trouble all the time with my work, I was going through the menopause, I was so tired. The feeling was overwhelming, I slept all the time, I couldn't concentrate, I could not do the job. Every task took me forever; I was so slow, I was forever dropping and breaking things, but I believed I was doing a good job and they were picking on me. They were always shouting at me, they thought I was lazy and I just could not do anymore. Continually I was getting called for more performance reviews. Why they didn't sack me- I do not know. They must have known that something was wrong? I asked if I could cut my shifts down and have more time off because I was too tired. They agreed, probably glad to get rid of me, but they let me use my holiday days so my pay was not affected. I had already taken big pay cuts with stepping down all the time. They kept dogging me to go to the Doctor's but when I had time off I was too tired. I just slept all the time, sometimes all day in my chair, I was completely exhausted.

I can only recall one Doctor's visit in May. I don't know what I told her but she had me walking up and down the surgery as though I was being breathalysed. Perhaps she thought I was an Alcoholic? She sent me for blood tests which came back that I was vitamin D and Calcium deficient and needed some sun, at least 20 minutes a day. That set my mind at rest that nothing was wrong, I had just been over doing things. My neighbour later told me that every sunny day I would sit on my bench in the sun for 20 minutes so that stuck in my mind. I carried on until I could not do anymore, my body was shutting down.

I started missing shifts, I could not get up, I didn't phone in and I knew after being a manager how important it is to let work know so your shift can be covered. I only wanted to sleep and couldn't be bothered anymore with anything and anybody. I stopped eating, drinking, and getting washed; it was all too much effort. I could have slept for a year and even then I didn't think I would have felt any different. I kept missing the bus, I had to have taxis every day, I just could not get moving but I still blamed everyone else. I didn't think it was me.

I had also developed a very bad pain in my left shoulder and found it difficult to raise my arm. I put it down to wear and tear with all the heavy work that I've done and, once again, age. I also had difficulty getting out of the bath as I just could not pull myself up. My daughter had to get me out on a few occasions after I had sat there for a long time waiting for her return, so I stopped having a bath and took to strip washes instead.

PERFORMANCE IMPROVEMENT PLAN

Employee's Name: Susan Jones   Position: Restaurant Team Member

Assessment date: 28th August 2014

Conducted by: ~~[redacted]~~

AREAS REQUIRING IMPROVEMENT	IMPROVEMENT REQUIRED	TRAINING REQUIRED
Speed and urgency	Perform all tasks at a faster pace	
Buffet set up	Increase speed of setting up the buffet to ensure that it is complete for the beginning of service	
Using the till	Able to take payments for breakfast	Till training
Interpreting breakfast reports	Able to understand and use breakfast reports	
Taking beverage orders	Able to take beverage orders and ensure that orders are delivered in a timely fashion.	
Communication with guests	Able to communicate with guests in a friendly and professional manner	
Sunday lunch service	Able to take orders, communicate with the kitchen and deliver the food to the correct standard and in a timely fashion	Sunday lunch service
Timekeeping	Improve rate of absenteeism and lateness. Follow procedure for absence reporting	

As discussed, if there is insufficient improvement seen by the required completion date of 11th September 2014, disciplinary action may be considered in respect of your poor performance.

I have read the above and agree with the assessment, comments and action arising. I agree with the review dates above

Employee's name ....

Employee's signature ... S. Jones .... Date 28/8/14

PERFORMANCE IMPROVEMENT PLAN

This was my last day worked as 14 days later I had major brain surgery, as you can see I was unable to perform very little. I then started to fall backwards without warning and could not get back up. I lost all power down my left side, I had to wait for people to pick me up, I cannot recall how many times but I was getting worried because I was losing my memory. I couldn't remember how I had fallen so people just thought I had tripped, and then I would just forget about it. Even though my memory was getting bad it didn't wipe out the awful pain in my arm so it must have been bad. My daughter was away a lot and I started feeling scared of being alone in case I fell.

It all came to a head on the 29th August 2014 when my daughter took me to the Doctor's as she thought I'd had a stroke. I couldn't raise my arm and I was having trouble speaking. When we got to see the doctor I did not know why I was there. In my mind there was nothing wrong with me and if I had gone alone I wouldn't have told him anything. According to my daughter he asked me why I had come and I replied; "I don't know". I cannot remember much of my visit and if she had not taken me and explained what was going on I would not be here today. I can only remember a couple of things which seemed strange. My daughter was telling him that I wasn't her mum as I now was a different person; I thought she was being disrespectful talking about me like that, I told her to be quiet. The doctor also looked in my eyes with a torch with the surgery lights off, I told him my eyesight was bad and that my left eye was the worst one, he said it "certainly was". Thanks to the Doctor's expertise, he had a suspicion it was a brain tumour and sent me for a C.T. scan. When I spoke to the Doctor at a later date he confirmed that I didn't tell him anything.

My memory would come and go which made it difficult for people to understand what was going on. I remember vividly the day before my C.T. scan which was a Sunday the 7th September 2014, I was bringing in my washing from the garden as I reached up with my left arm to unpeg it I was suddenly thrown backwards without warning and very quickly hit the path, I had no control over my body which was pretty terrifying at the time. I was paralyzed, no matter how hard I tried I just could not get myself up off the ground, lucky for me my neighbour had come out into his garden, we had a small wall separating us, he looked over and could see me laying in a heap of washing (what a sight?) "What are you doing?" he said "I've fallen and I cannot get up can you help me please?"

I replied. He shouted his nephew who was visiting at the time; they both jumped over the wall and stood me back up on my feet making a joke about it not realizing the seriousness of the fall. Stupid me said "don't worry I'm having a scan tomorrow" as if that made sense why I was on the ground. I had also wet myself probably with fear as I would have had to stay where I was until my daughter came home from the gym.

I went for my scan on the 8th September 2014 at the Northern General Hospital (not that I remember much about it). The only recollection I have is being put in a wheelchair and taken back to the clinic. I couldn't understand why I wasn't allowed to walk which was confusing as it was my arm that was the problem, not my legs. It still didn't register that it was my head. I thought it was my arm that was being scanned to see what was causing the terrible pain. I remember being told I would have to wait for an ambulance to take me to the Hallamshire Hospital as I was being transferred, I said, "don't worry I'll get a taxi." I still didn't understand and thought after my treatment I would be able to go home. It all happened so quickly, it really did not bother me. I was so confused. My daughter said I just laughed at everything they said. I was admitted as an emergency and cannot remember much about the start of my stay. I was sent for an MRI Scan and had needles stuck in my arm, my daughter told me that my consultant wouldn't let her look at the results as they were too horrific. I later found out from my daughter what happened in the hospital clinic.

The Chinese lady doctor had me doing some neurological tests like walking in a straight line to check my balance. I could not do this, I kept falling all over the place, laughing, she was getting annoyed with me when I could not follow her finger whilst keeping my head still. I thought she was nasty for shouting at me, so she asked a nurse to come over and hold my head still. My daughter said it was embarrassing. When we got back to the clinic after my scan the doctor could see why I wasn't able to perform her tasks and while speaking to her colleague on the phone she said this lady WALKED into my clinic this morning she was astounded! I should not have been walking with the size of the tumour in my head.

The operation to remove the tumour was scheduled for the 11th September. It was going to be a major operation that took 10 hours; it was growing in the lining of my brain on the left side at the front. I was extremely lucky that they could get at it and it wasn't attached-which saved me from both Chemotherapy and Radiotherapy. My surgeon managed to get it all out, it involved cutting my head open from ear to ear and pulling my face down and also smashing my skull. In effect, it was a face lift which some people pay thousands for. I was oblivious to all of this thank-goodness; we just had to wait to see if it was benign. The operation was a huge success and the news was good; it was benign. It was a Meningioma-a slow grower; it had been growing for about 20-30 years. It had reached an impressive golf ball size but according to my consultant it was the best type to have as it's the least aggressive. Now all I had to do was recover. After I came out of theatre and was put in recovery, my daughter and neighbour told me it was a very worrying time for them. They were talking to me when, suddenly, I did one loud snore and went into a deep sleep. The nurses and doctors could not wake me up. My daughter says they were cruel to me; sticking needles in my arms and legs, using the reflex hammer, tickling my feet, pulling the pipe in my neck and shouting my name, all to no avail. My neighbour says the male nurse at the bottom of the bed was looking at the monitor and saying it looked like I had had a seizure so they called my surgeon back in in case they had to operate again. They took me off to the C.T. scanner to see what was going on. It is quite common to have a bleed after such a major operation, thankfully that was not the case-it was the swelling, which was huge, that was threatening my life.

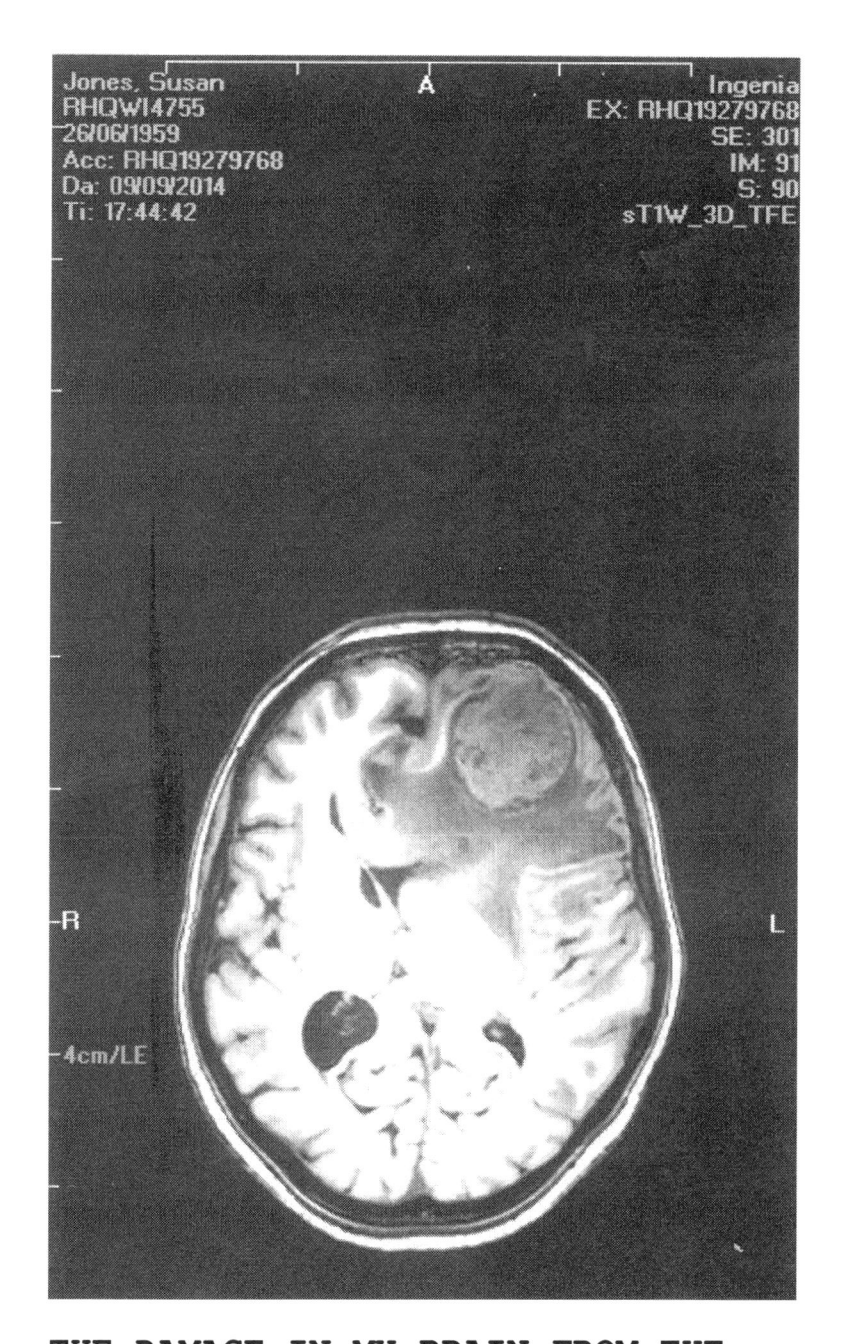

THE DAMAGE IN MY BRAIN FROM THE
MRI VIEW

My surgeon later told me he had just got home for tea with his family when he got a call about me. I apologized and he laughed and said that there was no way I was going to die on him after he had spent all those hours trying to save me. He was very pleased with his handy work of my staples and wanted to show them off; he eventually got home around midnight. What dedication! The surgeon and his team were brilliant! I will never be able to thank them enough, along with my neighbour, Doctor and Daughter, they saved my life.

When I went for my first check-up, my consultant told me that if the Doctor hadn't sent me for the scan when he did, I only had a short time left to live. The swelling in my brain was so bad that the left side had been pushed into the right side and my brain had actually bent to accommodate it. I'd also had a small seizure and when they re-scanned me the swelling was still the same and my brain had not gone back. I asked a few questions about recovery time, memory loss and the dreaded pain in my left arm. The recovery time was expected to be 9-12 months and two years for a full recovery.

Memory wise, what I don't get back after a year is as good as it gets and the arm pain was not connected to the tumour and needed investigating. It will be 10 years before I get the all clear and I will need regular scans. I also told him the drugs that I was given were awful, he replied, "Those drugs saved your life".

I was having bad headaches for a few years but my memory wiped away all the pain except for my left arm. I had told lots of people about the headaches so I must have been aware at the time. I remember going to have my eyes checked a couple of times in case my vision was the cause or my gas fire was faulty, both times different opticians called me back because they thought something was wrong but they never picked up on it, it's even on my records that I had complained of bad headaches at the back of my head.

My memory got so bad I don't really know what I've been doing, friends and relations have been filling me in on how I've been behaving and a lot makes sense now. I was falling asleep everywhere, home, when I went to visit my mum, the works canteen. I wasn't aware of this. I was repeatedly asking people the same questions over and over again, I was confused, I forgot people's names, work colleagues who I had worked with for a long time, I started living in the past and going back in time, friends, neighbours, relations say I was vacant and looked through them as if I didn't comprehend. My work colleagues stopped talking to me; I probably frustrated them and scared them. This upset me because I couldn't understand why? People avoided me and I tried frantically to find another job but I was too tired to chase them up. My work colleagues thought I was depressed, or was having a mental breakdown or I was getting the signs of early senile dementia. I was a different person. I stopped going out, I lost contact with friends, never answered my phone, letters. They knew something wasn't right, they would call at my door but I never answered, I was either at work or asleep. The signs were there but they were never acted upon. When my employers found out what was wrong with me I asked my close colleagues if they had known that something wasn't right? Yes they knew. I wasn't the same person as when I first started working for them. I didn't work in the same way, they thought I was sulking and lazy because I wasn't doing what was asked of me, but more and more work was piled on top of me. I couldn't go any faster and was always late finishing my shift, I wasn't performing to standards. They kept sending me home and telling me to go to the Doctor's.

I wasn't aware of this; I must have been a nightmare to work with. What I needed was someone to take me to the Doctors and explain how I was behaving although it wouldn't have made much difference- the damage was already done; I was very near the end. I was always ok health wise so I never went to the Doctors. I was just too busy to be ill; I just got on with it.

As my memory is now slowly coming back a lot of things I was doing at work now makes sense. I wondered why I could never carry the milk jugs without tipping it all down me when all the other staff managed. I must have been losing my balance.

I even recall asking for a full apron as my blouse was always soaked. I also recall doing the floor run where you had to collect all the previous evenings' room service trays with crockery and glasses, I never got them back to the kitchen without breakages, they would slip off the trolley. I blamed the fire doors and the lift for catching them when it was obviously me. I also recall not being able to deliver the room service breakfast's without spilling the drinks all over the trays no matter how careful I walked. We laugh about this now but it wasn't funny at the time. I was a complete nightmare. I also have a vague memory of not being able to set tables for breakfast and dinner no matter how many times I was shown, but in my mind I believed my set up was correct and it was others that could not do it, I even remember some little photographs being placed on the serving station for me to look at, my manager later told me I was very hard work, one day I would set up fine and the next day I had no idea what to do, she would ask if I had got my photo's. I just did not have a clue what she was on about and she could not work out what was wrong with me. Now that my memory is almost back, I am obsessed with the set-up of tables, as should I fall ill again, I don't want anyone to think it's me.

2.

MY JOURNEY TO RECOVERY

I suppose you could say it started on the 12th of September 2014, not that I know much about it as I was too ill and drugged up. My daughter and family and friends have been filling me in and some of my memory is now returning, I will never know the full story but I can only piece together what I've been told. I was on lots of strong drugs which were going to have me climbing the walls by the end, according to what the surgeon told my daughter. They had to get the swelling down, otherwise I wouldn't survive. I was placed in critical care, but I wasn't aware of this. It was the most frightening experience of my life and I hope I never have to go through that again. To me, it was very real and I thought I was trapped in a horrible world. I believed the hospital was evil and the people were trying to kill me, they were chopping patients up at night and putting them in body bags to dispose of them. I must have been given a higher dose at night and I dreaded nightfall, I kept trying to escape and wouldn't stay in bed, the everyday noises and the equipment played a part in my nightmare. I was watched carefully as I was placed next to the nurse's station. Although in my mind, (it was screwed up) was the hotel reception, I thought I was going mad. The staff knew what the drugs were going to do to me so were used to it. I believed they were trying to stop me escaping. My name was first on the patient's board so when the staff changed shift in the evening they would discuss what I had been given, but I was so screwed up when I heard my name, I panicked and thought, shit! It's my turn. There was no way I was going to sleep, I needed to stay awake. I had to get out of there fast; it was like a horror movie. Why would my daughter leave me in a place like this? I phoned my daughter and best friend in the middle of the night telling them that they wouldn't see me anymore. I told them that I loved them and goodbye, I suppose I sounded frantic, but also realistic and frightening.

We laugh about this now but it was awful at the time. I also upset my mum by phoning and telling her they were throwing me out as they needed the bed. My mum believed me, but no way was that going to happen, not a couple of days after a major operation. My daughter also tells me that I called her in the middle of the night and told her to come and fetch me because they were throwing me out. If she didn't come, I would have to stay on the town hall steps. My daughter laughs about this. She said I would have been easily recognized with a big bandage on my head and two black eyes! I remember being very cunning (or so I thought). I watched the other patients to see what they did and tried to work out my escape plan. There was another lady who had the same name as me and was roughly my age that always got up in the night, she would go to the nurses station and ask for a cup of tea. They would leave her there while they went and made her one. Great! I thought, that's what I will do, and while they are not watching me, I can get out of the place. However, it didn't work for me, they escorted me back to my bed and brought the tea to me, they didn't miss a thing. I also recall getting the lady involved in my nightmare, I believed the nurses were police women and they were going to section me because I'd gone mad. They went to the other lady by mistake, who hadn't a clue what was going on, I shouted and told them "it's me, not her!" and that I knew what they were up to! They must have had a good laugh about this afterwards, although they will have seen this behaviour many times. I was asked if I was going to hurt myself or did I want to hurt anyone else, the drugs must have had me hallucinating. I don't remember the outcome, although I can recall a nurse telling other staff that I had gone mad. It was like going to hell and back. I was also confused over why I couldn't find my clothes and I had to keep asking for a gown. My daughter later told me that the hospital contacted her and asked if I had any outdoor clothes. They were aware that I was trying to do a runner. I kept asking my friend to bring me some clothes and they kept taking them, they took all my belongings and tagged them, kept them secure until I was discharged. I would have been spotted more easily in a hospital gown, especially as I couldn't put them on properly and had the nurses running after me as I was exposed. It was a mixed ward but we all had neurological problems. I must have been hard work for the poor hospital staff. It was a very frightening experience, one I don't think I will ever forget.

My mum also told me that every time she came to visit me, I wasn't in bed. I was sat on the edge, fully clothed, no wonder they wanted me in a gown. She also said one time I wasn't in my ward she found me further down wearing another patients footwear. I told her mine were too slippy and I was being bossy and telling other visitors, "only one to a bed". They weren't even visiting me! I cannot recall any of this. I do remember saying to my consultant that "I'm not a person that sits still". He replied, "I know that".

I also remember a couple of surreal experiences as I was coming down off the drugs, I remember waking up in the middle of the night as though I was laying on a slab completely alone and looking up at bright lights. It was deathly silent, peaceful, and I thought I'd died. The noises in my head had stopped, I later found out that it was the nerve endings that had been severed and were firing off. I also remember a chaplain coming to see me before the operation and asking if they could include me in their evening prayers and ask god to see me through this difficult time. I also remember waking up one morning and not knowing who the people at the bottom of my bed were, it was the surgeon and his team, I didn't know where I was and what were they doing this to me for, I wouldn't obey and told them to leave me alone, they took blood out of me and two nurses dragged me crying for a shower to wake me up. It must have been the come down. It's funny how you remember the bad things.

Before I could get discharged I had to be able to walk up and down stairs, my bathroom and bedroom are located upstairs. I suppose I could have used a commode and have a bed of some kind brought downstairs until I was fit and well again but the hospital physio's were relentless pushing you every day I kept losing my balance so they got me a walking stick. That was a farce at first, I kept falling over the damn thing and it was supposed to help me! I also had to be able to get something to eat and drink so they put me in a wheelchair and took me to a mock-up kitchen in the basement of the hospital to teach me how to make a hot drink and some toast. I had no idea how to use a toaster having never had one, so I wouldn't be doing that when I got home. I couldn't get my balance, never mind find my way round a strange kitchen. I had just had Brain surgery for goodness sake! I suppose with living alone they didn't want me to starve to death.

3.

COMING HOME

I remember coming home in a taxi with my daughter, it was very nerve wracking, I had been in hospital for 11 days and it had all happened so fast. Two nurses were waiting for me, as they had to assess my home to see if I was safe and what my needs would be. I didn't even recognise my home; I was so confused as it was very dirty. It couldn't be mine! Nothing worked; no lights, water, and it was full of dust. I don't know how I'd been living, I was too ill to care. I had had a long day waiting to be discharged, it was tea-time, and I was tired and I needed my bed. I was also very afraid of being left alone without the security of the hospital in case anything went wrong.

I had a care team who came every day for a month to help me with physio and to check on me to see what I needed to make my life easier. They organized a bath seat which was fitted for me and they performed memory tests and checked my health. My daughter sorted out a system with the drugs so that all I had to do was take them, it worked well. The pain was terrible even though I was still taking lots of medication, it didn't seem to do any good. I couldn't sleep as my head was too sore to lie on. My left arm I could have cheerfully chopped off! I had extremely bad nightmares when I did drop off, and panic attacks, and I would often wake up sobbing. I didn't know why I just couldn't stop. I sometimes had dark thoughts-that I would rather not wake up if this was going to be what my life was going to be like, but my surgeon wouldn't have been pleased after all his hard work to save me. I still have a lot of pain today, but I've learnt to cope with it and it's nowhere near as bad.

PHOTO'S OF MY RECOVERY AT HOME

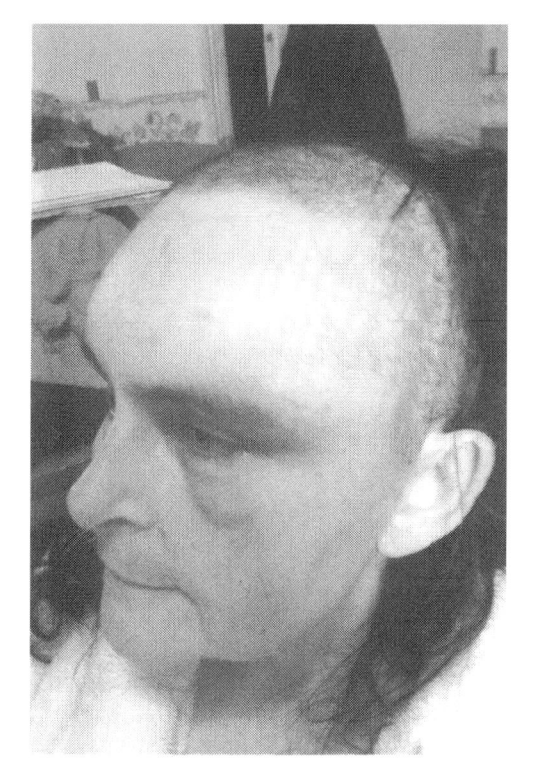

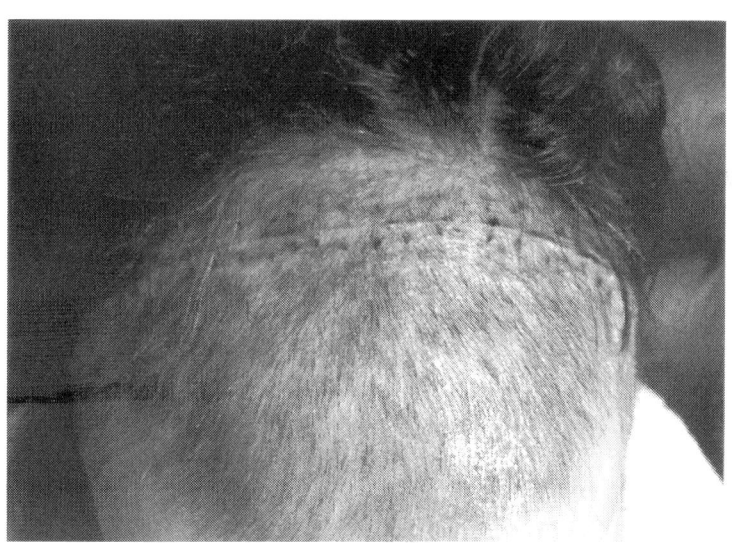

The Brilliant art work from my surgeon

My bruised and swollen face

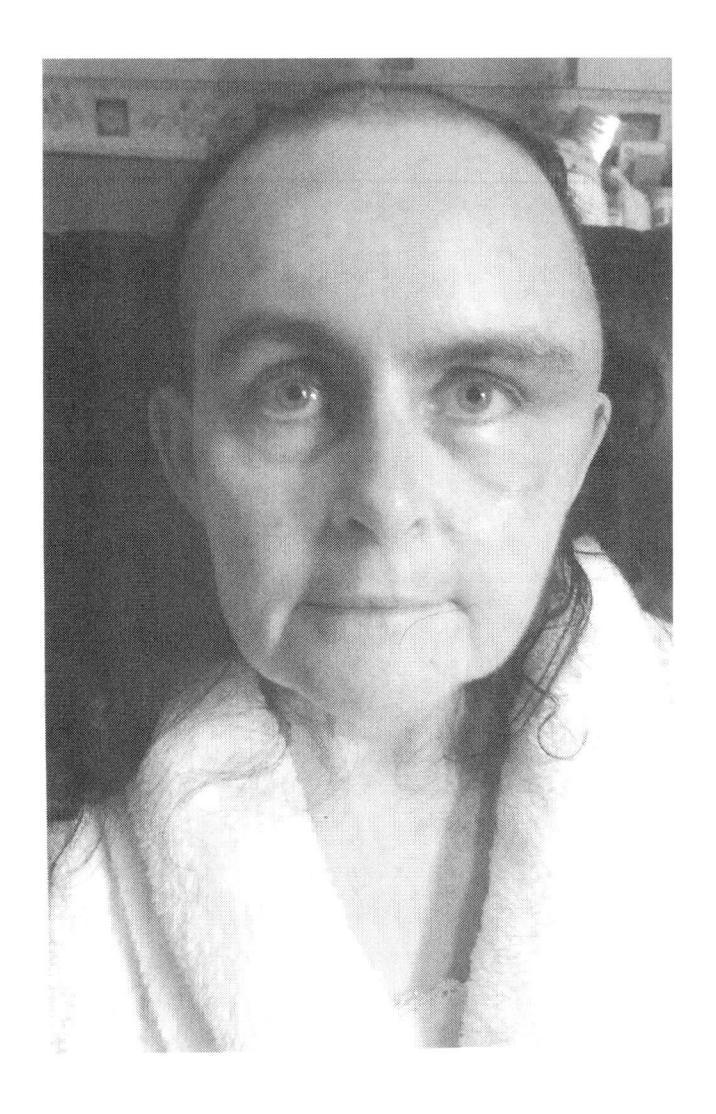

I had to learn everyday basic things like putting on my gas fire and cooker, I struggled with the fire. My good friend and her husband came and sorted out my lights and water which was great and made it much safer. I was unsteady on my feet and had very bad dizzy spells, which was alien to me and very nerve racking. I was lucky to live in a small house, so there was always plenty of furniture to hold on to. I had great friends and neighbours, who came every day between them to check on me, bought me meals, did my shopping, along with my daughter, and offered their support. I'm so lucky to have such wonderful friends and family who helped me through, I don't know what I would have done without them.

I am an independent person who has faced many challenges and I don't like asking for help, I find it hard not to be in control, I'm used to being the one that helps others.

My care team consisted of a great guy and two therapists. The guy was a physio who put me through my paces and, when I got stronger, took me out into the big wide world for a walk. I used his arm and my stick, it was weird. We continued until I was confident to let go of his arm and just use my stick, he still walked at my side as I still swayed. My daughter also took me for walks in between when the weather was ok. My friends and neighbours also cheered me up and we would laugh about my antics, which I didn't know of, in the hospital. My daughter recalled what I said to the medical team in response to their questions. When asked what year it was I replied, "1997," without hesitation and, "who was the prime minister?" I said "Gordon Brown." With later research, Gordon Brown was indeed prime minister in 1997, so I had gone back in time. It must have been a good year for me to go back to, I still haven't found out why yet though. I also remember them asking me questions all the time such as; did I know where I was? "Yes" I replied, "the Hallamshire hotel," I just couldn't think of it as a hospital, a hotel and a hospital are very similar with having beds and lots of people rushing around. I think they gave up on me with that one, my daughter did say the surgeon asked her what I did for a living and that explained it. I also recall the question, "Can you count backwards from 100 in 7's?" I couldn't even count forwards! That question haunted me and I got all my friends, family and neighbours to have a go when I was home and back in reality. I still cannot do it to this day. I got all my visitors mixed up and called them each other's names; I told them any old rubbish. My daughter and sister asked me what I'd had for dinner. I replied, "Tuna and stuffing sandwiches." Where I got that one from I don't know, maybe I might try it one day. I couldn't operate my mobile phone and I sent lots of strange and unreadable messages, my mind just couldn't fathom how to do it. My daughter said she was relieved when my credit ran out. I obviously wasn't, I couldn't understand why it wasn't working anymore and I ended up deleting all the numbers. Then, I was trapped in this horrible place with no contact to the outside world; my worst nightmare.

I have met some really lovely people who have helped me on my journey and who do a great job. I've had lots of ups and downs, severe pain, loss, emotions, anger and frustrations. As I got stronger, my daughter took me further to the shops and the bank. I had to learn how to do all these tasks again. I found it hard with the bank machines as I couldn't remember how to use them and I couldn't recall my pin number. My daughter wrote everything down in a little notebook. The staff in the local supermarket was fantastic, they all knew me as I had shopped there for the past 30 years, they all helped me to find items and help me pay for them. It was like starting again and I got frustrated a lot and felt useless when I couldn't do things. I'm not a very patient person at the best of times and can be very stubborn. I made it out into the big wide world on my own in late October, just to the local shop. It was very challenging and scary and I was panicky. I still had balance issues and my walking stick plus, I had a very bad fear of main roads. I was slow and traffic was fast, so I had to use the side roads and crossings, but I made it. Once I got started there was no stopping me and I set myself goals to go further and further. I did overdo it quite often and it would set me back a few days, but you cannot keep me grounded. The first time I crossed a main road without a crossing was the end of March, it took me a long time and was very daunting I had to wait for a long gap before I plucked up the courage. I'm still very careful today.

I'd still got the nasty shoulder and arm pain so I went to seek medical advice. I was sent for an x-ray and an ultrasound to find out the problem, my GP didn't know whether I'd damaged it when I was falling or if I'd got Ostia-arthritis. When I got my results it was diagnosed as a frozen shoulder. I was sent for physio and it's still ongoing although the pain is not as bad, I just cannot raise my arm fully as it's locked. It can take a few years to heal and because I over used my right arm to compensate I developed Tennis elbow which is also very painful and needs rest and physio so I'm armless. I decided to keep a diary to record my goals and my achievements as it also helps me with my memory and to chart my recovery. I've met some wonderful people who I can never repay who have supported me financially who without them I would have had a slower recovery, I am so grateful; they have been there for me in my hours of need.

The first time I went on a bus alone was January 2015. Everything seemed so daunting as we take things for granted. I was very pleased with myself and, like a child, I wanted to plan another journey and go further. I had a lot of set-backs when the weather turned bad, the ice was a problem so I was back to being housebound, but, as soon as it was safe, I was itching to get back out. The first time I went without my stick was late February 2015. It was scary, I had dizzy spells and overbalanced but I did it and didn't look back. If I have a dizzy spell now, which is quite often, I just stand still until it passes and if I overbalance I just grab the nearest thing, it will get better with time although I do still panic. I could not do a lot of things that I used to love doing, it was either too painful or I'd forgotten how to. I loved reading but it hurt my head and I couldn't remember what I had read so it seemed a waste of time, but by doing little and often, it has improved. I'm not very good at retaining information, if the story is too deep and boring, so I try to go for light reading and captivating storylines. I joined the local library and started with large print books so as not to hurt my head as much and now I can read almost anything-only for short sessions though. I've also had to learn how to spell again, my spelling was atrocious. I could see it looked wrong but I couldn't remember the correct way, so I've used an old dictionary which fortunately I'd kept and used to write this story. I couldn't remember how to do simple maths such as adding up and subtracting, I was useless and spent many hours checking my finances, I now use a calculator but I still double check and write everything down. I've also had to learn how to use my mobile phone, texting was a problem. It was shocking and the messages I did send were unreadable, but with practise I've got better. It hurts my head to use a handset so I had to learn fast so I could communicate with the outside world. I've also taken up the opportunity to go on a free basics computer course at the local library with a tutor who is very patient with me. I had completely forgotten how to use one but I am now sending E-mails with the help of my note book. I've also made some new friends and learnt a new skill. Each time I achieve one goal, I get more confident although sometimes I get frustrated have lots of tears, get angry with myself and feel useless, which in turn makes my pains worse. I've just got to be patient and, with time, things will improve. The first time I went out of my comfort zone was the beginning of May 2015, I had pondered about doing this for a few weeks after my friend had taken me in her car; I did some research about where the bus stops were and which bus to catch and how to get back, it was to visit Crystal Peaks shopping centre. It was unfamiliar territory and I panicked over what if when I get off the bus there is a main road without a safe place to cross. What will I do? It was a daunting journey and I didn't really enjoy it. I had bad pains in my head and felt sick, probably nerves more than anything, I started thinking I had come too far and I needed to go back but I carried on and achieved what I had set out to do, it was the furthest I had travelled alone. I haven't gone any further since and I used to travel all over the place alone, it's just trying to build my confidence, which I am sure I will in time.

I have still got a long way to go and I will naturally have lots of setbacks. I have just got to adapt to my new circumstances and learn to realise that I will not be able to do what I used to do, but I can learn new skills and different ways around things. The most important thing is that I am alive and I have had a second chance, I am so lucky and blessed it could have been such a very different story. It puts things into perspective-that life is precious and too short –so live every day to the full. I have still got lots more learning and challenges to overcome and I may never get all my memory back but today starts from now.

It is now the 11th of September, one year on, and I have still got a long way to go and a lot more to learn. It has been very hard, painful, emotional and madly stressful, but I am on my way to getting back to some normality and the start of my new life, so it is all positive. It has been a life changing experience and has brought back all my old friends who I had lost contact with because of being too busy and I have made many new friends along my journey.

It has also taught me not to judge people as no one knows what goes on in their lives and just because they look well does not mean they are not in a lot of pain. Now I have had to slow down it is amazing all the things that I have missed by being too busy, I never had the time to watch nature, the birds taking the seeds and the pampas grass to feather their nests and the beautiful colours and the scents of the plants and the flowers as the seasons change. The dawn chorus of the birds, and the owls hooting at night, it really is amazing. If it had not been for my brain tumour I would have missed all this, so I really should have said thank you.

I have been for my first MRI scan since my operation to see if everything's ok, my consultant is very pleased with the results and thinks that I am making a remarkable recovery. The swelling has abated and the left side of my brain has gone back to where it should be. He did not expect it to go back so quickly, so it's the best news he could have hoped for. He's also pleased that I have not had any more seizures. It's very reassuring. I remember when I had to start decreasing the anti-convulsants, I felt safe while I was on them, but halving the first dose I was told if I had a fit it would occur in the first seven days. That was ok as my daughter was still living with me, but coming off them completely and if I had another one within 3 months was frightening as I was alone. I was afraid of banging my head if I fell. I have got another scan in March 2016 so at least they will keep an eye on me, so onwards and upwards!

The horrendous journey of my recovery started when I got discharged from hospital as the people I expected to support me let me down. Starting with my employers, they could only give me statutory sick pay instead of company sick pay even though they had the means and the final say. It didn't matter that I had worked for the company for the past five years, I never had time off sick, I did above and beyond, worked long, long hours which I didn't get paid for as I was salaried. You were supposed to take it back in time but there never was any spare time, but I never complained because I took it all on myself as I loved my job. It was exceptional circumstances, after all, but it made no difference, that was the policy for all employees no matter what. I needed their support but it didn't happen. I was just a number, statutory sick pay as everyone knows is peanuts and very hard to live on and it was more stress I did not need. I had just undergone a major brain operation and was seriously ill.

I was not entitled to anything from the state as I had my own home with the help of a mortgage which was still on going, but fortunately for me I had taken out mortgage payment protection which covered my main mortgage for 12 months should anything happen to me to stop me paying my monthly repayments. This too was a problem as I needed a medical certificate to get it released and I could not afford the £60 so I had to use my credit card. Thank God I had back-up. I also had to use my credit card to live on and for my medication which was £8 a prescription, everything had to be paid for. I was in tremendous pain, alone, I was not very good at communicating, I was hitting brick walls all the time when I was supposed to be recovering, I could not get out as I was unsteady on my feet, very fearful and I had very dark thoughts. I was totally at rock bottom.

Things got much worse as the months went on, I got into a lot of debt with no way of repaying it until I could get well and get back to work. No one would help me. I cut down as much as I could; I lived in one room with one gas fire (which was dodgy). I don't have central heating and I wouldn't have been able to afford it anyway. I did not need much food so I lived mostly on noodles and toast. I was too ill to care, I budgeted £5 a week for food and I did manage on it with the help of my mum (she's a pensioner) my neighbour and carer and my best friend, they gave me food parcels, home grown vegetables and salad and also cooked an extra portion of their stews and chillies. I hated feeling vulnerable; I don't like asking for help as I am a very proud person. I can put on a brave face but, behind closed doors, I was heartbroken. How was I going to get through all this? Would it not have been better if I had died during the operation? I know it is ungrateful and that life is precious, but this was a living hell. There were days when I would get my fighting spirit back and try to be positive but the bad days outweighed the good, I had to push myself to get stronger so I could get back to work and not because I liked the place anymore, it caused me lots of nightmares, but it was a means to an end.

Winter set in and more misery came my way as my gas fire broke. This left me without any heating at all. My neighbour had bought herself a new oil filled radiator which she kindly let me borrow until I could get a gas fitter to come, that weekend was the coldest on record and I froze. Next came Christmas and it was a very miserable one for me I could not give presents and I felt useless when friends and family bought me gifts of food parcels and food vouchers so that I could have a little cheer but I could not give back. Why me? I felt so low and embarrassed; I promised myself that I would repay everyone when I was back on my feet.

Things started getting a little better again and I had more hope. Word had got out about what had happened to me and my former employers were very worried. They managed to get me a hospitality grant and a top up payment for the next 12 months, it was not a great amount but it was the world to me and without it I would have gone under, I would probably have had to sell my home and I was not well enough to even attempt that.

Then my statutory sick pay ended and I was placed on Employment support allowance. What a joke, £73 a week? I wasn't being ungrateful but it was even less than the statutory sick pay. On the upside, at least I could rely on getting paid and not have to worry if work had forgotten to pay me again, which had happened on a few occasions. I was now also entitled to apply for pip (personal independence payment) from the Department of works and pensions. I had to go for a consultation which they sent me to a place I had never been, I had no transport, I was unsteady on my feet, it was early days in my recovery and I was very nervous. This was totally unacceptable, but if I did not go my benefit would stop. I got ever so upset over this and my dear friend stepped in once again, her husband took the day off work and they took me, I don't know what I would have done without them, this was unnecessary-I'm sure it could have been done in my home town. Needless to say, I didn't qualify after all, I was truly devastated, it was all for nothing-just a lot of stress which I did not need.

4.

REHABILITATION

I have started going to a Brain and Head injury rehabilitation centre. The first time I went to the centre alone, I was extremely anxious and had to plan my route because I needed to work out where I could cross the roads safely. It was in an unfamiliar area, it really took it out of me and it was very demanding. It was ok at first, but then I had to incorporate bus fares, it was four buses for one appointment and the sessions were two to three a week to start with, as I had to see lots of different Therapists. This was seriously eating into my food money and I was getting more distressed. I asked the centre to try and put my sessions all on one day where possible to make it easier for me, they couldn't do it all the time as they have lots of patients and they all have individual needs. I have met lots of lovely people who work there, an Occupational therapist, Physiotherapist, Speech therapist and a Psychologist. At first I was not sure why I needed to see all these people and I was being stubborn, I thought I was ok. I know best, and I don't need help, I can do it all on my own, so I fought against them. I got angry and ended up losing my temper until I went away and spoke to friends, family and realised they were only trying to help me and I needed their support. After I calmed down and got to know these people, I felt less vulnerable and opened up more, I apologized for my outburst understanding that they were only trying to do their jobs. I was just frustrated. They tried to help me get a bus pass and also help with my prescription charges as I wasn't getting them, I had to buy the cheaper versions, but they were not doing the correct job. I was getting ill, it was a choice of pills or food, I was in pain and had even more health issues. My goal and with their help was to be able to return to work, that in itself was going to be an enormous challenge. I am excited but apprehensive, I have got a lot to re-learn and I don't want to look silly but I've got great support from my therapists at the centre.

I went to the Brain injury Rehabilitation Centre for about 18 months, sometimes I would come away and feel that it was all a waste of time, and other times I would try to take on board the things that were suggested I try to make my life easier; after all they are the experts. We had lots of issues to work through to get me back to fitness, some were very challenging, especially when I was not well, I suffered with vertigo which can be triggered as part of a brain injury and can be terrifying as you lose your balance and get very dizzy. I also suffered with fatigue. I'm not one for stopping or slowing down so I found this most disappointing at times. Some of the physio was mind blowing even if you've not just had brain surgery, to stand and stare at a spot on the door and move your head left to right to see how dizzy you are? Or if you lose your balance? It would have made more sense to go on the waltzer at the fairground? It felt like I was shaking what was left in my head out! But hey! I don't know what my neighbours thought I was doing when practicing at home it probably just confirmed to them that I had gone mad!

It got even worse when I got to walking up and down the large gym-type treatment room. Moving my head left to right and not looking down at the floor, trying to avoid objects that had been placed all around, this was to replicate my job as a breakfast waitress (who on earth walks around like that in a normal world?) It was to try and stop me from looking down all the time, but if it got me better who am I to complain? No wonder I had vertigo though. Little did I know at the time that I had another small growing tumour in there? Without the support of the centre I would not have got back to work with the help I needed as my therapists liaised with my Employers and we all had a couple of meetings to discuss my needs. They had a look round my place of work for any potential hazards and kept in touch with the Human Resource Manager for an update on my progress, I liked having the safety net.

My mortgage payment protection was coming to an end and I still was not fit for work, this brought further stress. The department of work and pensions (DWP) had sent me a letter saying they would take over the interest payments on the mortgage. Until, they dropped a bombshell that I was not now entitled to it anymore. That's when I nearly gave up, I got so depressed, my therapists, family and friends were very worried about me. I could not pay a mortgage out of my income as well, it was not possible. I decided that my only option was to run up my credit card to pay my bills. I didn't really want to do this after my best friends husband had paid it all off once and allowed me to pay a small monthly payment of what I could afford; no matter how long it took, to help me get back on my feet. It felt as though I was throwing his kindness back in his face. I wanted to cancel anymore treatment and go back to work full-time, even though I knew deep down I was not well enough and I wouldn't be able to sustain it. I didn't know what else to do and, to top it all off, the Hospitality grant was coming to an end. Things were getting worse. I just wanted to go to my bed, get under the duvet and never get up. My occupational therapist tried her best to get me help by contacting Debt Agencies like Shelter and Step Change and making appointments for me to try and solve or put a period of time on my out-goings. I was not really in a fit state to be doing all this and found it very demeaning, filling in all the questions and speaking to them about all my financial mess. It made me feel that I had brought all this on by having a Brain Tumour, it was my own fault. They even suggested we would have to go to court to sort out my mess. I was horrified. I just could not do this! They even tried to get me access to a food bank. Just when I thought things could not get any worse, a glimmer of hope presented itself when I discovered my Life Insurance Policy while searching through my papers for details which had a critical illness cover with it that I had taken out in case I became ill, with being a single parent with a mortgage many years ago, upon closer inspection the claim had to be made 6 months after the brain tumour which had expired so my hopes were dashed again but I decided to try I had nothing to lose and I was desperate. I had lost my memory with the tumour so I didn't even know that I had a life policy, my surgeon and doctor confirmed this in writing and to my greatest surprise in the new year it was granted my mortgage was paid off! That was fantastic news and all my other worries were now not as important as I had a roof over my head. No matter what anything else got thrown at me, I could recover, which I hadn't otherwise been allowed to do.

Even though I have lots of health issues I am now back at work, only 6 hours a week at the moment. My therapists were right I would not have been able to do anymore but to save my sanity I would have tried.

5.

LIFE GOES ON

APRIL 2016

After starting back at work I noticed that I was having problems with breathlessness, palpitations and chest pain when I got exerted so I went to see my GP to get it checked out. I was probably doing too much too soon and my body needed to adjust, she sent me for an ECG (electrocardiogram) at the local hospital. When I received my results there was a problem so an appointment was made to see a Cardiologist all in the space of 2 weeks. It was very frightening to think I now might have problems with my heart what else could go wrong?

When I got to see Mr. B the Cardiologist he performed another ECG and did an examination I asked him if the ECG was ok this time, "I'm afraid not it's got blips on it" I am going to refer you for some heart scans at the Northern General Hospital. Blips? What on earth are those?

At the end of May, I went for the first part of the nuclear scan; they prodded and poked me then injected a dose of Radiation and sent me back to the scanner where I had to wait for 2 hours. This was scary and it seemed to be full of older people. Had they got this wrong? After I had the scan, which made me very fearful, it showed a problem, so I had to wait another half an hour and have it repeated. Only me, everyone else sailed through. It was exhausting. I wasn't allowed to eat or drink since the evening before, only a sip of water after a bad reaction to the stress test. What a day! I had to repeat this all again the following week, part 2, the only good thing was I now knew what to expect but without the Radiation this time, I couldn't believe my own bad luck when this scan had problems also and I had to have it repeated. The following week, I had to go to a different part of the hospital for an ultrasound on my heart. This one was a breeze in comparison and all I had to do now was wait for the results.

I was called back to see the cardiologist at the end of August. Everything is wait, wait, wait! It's a good job my GP had started me on medication, my results showed that my heart was working normally, it was just stiff? I asked him to explain. I wanted to laugh you hear the term being a stiff it was just nerves. The bottom part of my heart had calcified and I had slight hardening of the arteries, "Clinical Angina" I was to stay on the medication for life with regular checks, he even upped my dosage. I've since been diagnosed with Coronary heart disease which was probably caused by having a major operation on my brain. I also asked what the blips meant on my ECG-it signals heart trouble.

SEPTEMBER 2016

It is now two years since I had my operation to remove my brain tumour, unfortunately I also have another small one on the top of my head in the centre, it is in the lining of my brain it's the same type and it's not growing or causing me any problems, hopefully it never will and at least this time I know it exists.

My surgeon is happy with my recovery and we have agreed that after my next scan next year if everything is ok we can leave the scanning for 2 years, if I feel unwell or have any problems I can always contact him so things are moving on.

I have also been discharged from the head injury rehabilitation centre which is also great news.

I am still having problems with my health and I still have good days and bad days, I probably always will. I have got some normality back in my life, my memory has improved and I am learning lots of new skills. My confidence is returning and I've even been put forward for an award for exceptional customer service in my job which is a great achievement in such a short space of time. I am working more hours and even having a little social life, I have still got to push myself to go further afield it's just getting out of your comfort zone, small steps and I will make it.

MY EXCEPTIONAL CUSTOMER SERVICE AWARD

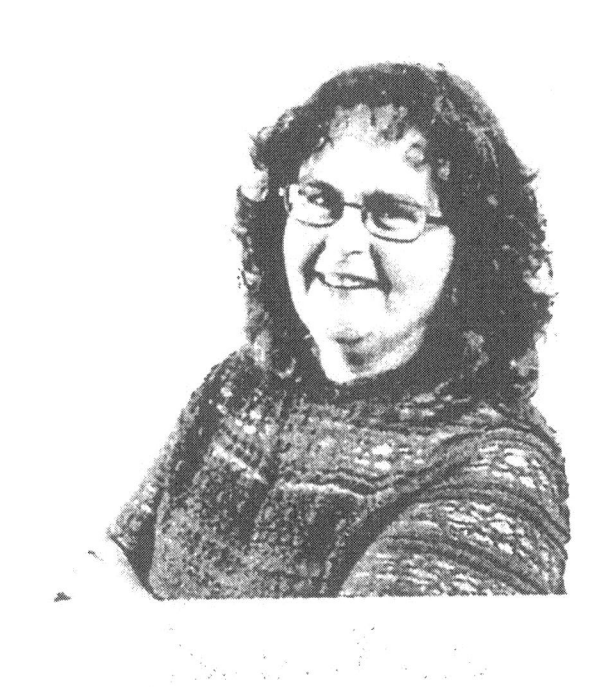

BREAKFAST WAITRESS

OCTOBER 2016

While I was recovering I decided to start a little project I don't know where I got little from? I was so ashamed of the state of my bedroom when the NHS were caring for me that it was time to have a go at decorating it, I had not done this for a few years, I was always working and never had any spare time. I thought it would take my mind off things and give me something positive to aim for; it was also a good excuse to have a huge clear-out.

It took me a good two months to paint and wallpaper and at times I felt like giving up I thought I had made a massive mistake, the furniture was heavy to move, my strength was not 100% I was still dizzy especially when climbing the ladder, my neighbour kept coming round to see if I was still in one piece but I am not a person who gives in so after a stern talking to myself I carried on and got the job done. I could not believe I had completely decorated a room all on my own. I was so proud I even treated myself to a new carpet to finish it off. How I managed to get the old one out I still cannot fathom.

SEPTEMBER 2017

It is now September 2017, nearly 3 years since my brain tumour operation. It has, so far, been a very eventful year. I went for my yearly mri scan in April to check on my meningioma's, the original one is not growing back, which is good news, but unfortunately the small one has been growing for the past 3 years which was a shock. Here we go again? It is scary information especially when I was told it was not doing anything, I needed to see my consultant as I had lots of questions to ask him I wanted reassurance that I was going to be ok? It was all positive news, I asked him why he hadn't told me sooner he thought it might stop growing of its own accord but that seems unlikely, I asked him what he would do in my position he replied "leave well alone, just get on with your life and don't worry." I am well at the moment and it's not affecting me, we have decided to do the "watch and wait" with yearly scans to monitor its growth, as long as it continues to grow slowly it should get me 10 years before it causes me problems.

We have opted for Stereotactic Radiosurgery which should hopefully stop it growing if successful, I trust my surgeon to know what is best for me, and after all he saved my life.

Stereotactic Radiosurgery is something I am not looking forward to it sounds very scary, it is a high dose of Radiation which is delivered in one single shot, my head will be placed in a frame which in itself sounds horrific, they drill 4 holes in your head under anaesthetic. Two are placed in the front of your head and two in the back of your skull, you are then placed in a machine similar to a mri scanner but without the noise for about 2 hours, imagine not being able to move for that length of time? At least with surgery you are put under, it's the recovery that takes its toll. The tumour is in a difficult place to reach for my consultant to do surgery and I don't really want to go through this again, everything has side effects it is a chance you have to take and at least it is not as invasive, with all the research something new could be out there by then. My only downfall is I could develop more tumours its just chance! Unless a miracle happens and the tumour stops growing of its own accord? I have already asked this question and it seems unlikely.

I am trying to just live my life and fill every day, sometimes I have dark thoughts that I'm going to die it's only natural, it is a weird feeling that something is growing inside your head, until you have experienced it you cannot judge.

I am now working 4 days a week and I love my job it keeps me sane (if there is such a thing) I laugh a lot and enjoy everything I attempt even though I cannot always get it right, I've still got a lot of hurdles to overcome. I will never forget this journey, it has been the hardest of my life so far but I can now see the light at the end of the tunnel which I never thought would happen.

ACKNOWLEDGEMENTS

I would like to say a special thank you to a few people who have helped me along my journey.

I cannot even begin to thank the wonderful NHS staff from Consultants, Theatre staff, Radiographers, Nurses, Physio's, Cleaners and everyone else who took great care of me on my unexpected journey without your skills and expertize I would not be here today, you do a most rewarding job.

Thanks to all my dearest friends, neighbours, family and therapists who without I would not have got through this difficult time as quickly, especially my amazing friend and neighbour who has been more like my carer and confidant and who checks on me every day. Thank you to my best friend for her support and with whom I have laughed and cried. Also the Hospitality Action Charity who have supported me and taken some of the stresses away, thank you so much.

I must also mention my daughter for designing the Book Cover exactly as I wanted it and for putting up with my criticism when things didn't work out.

Anyone else who I have not mentioned, you know who you are, I am so grateful for your caring and understanding patience.

Last but not least my wonderful friend Laura Huntley author of
The Black Eyed Boy who has dedicated her time to proof-read my work and pointed me in the right direction for which I am grateful for.

My Crazy Cell Mate - Susan Jones

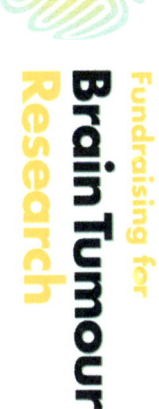

Fundraising for Brain Tumour Research

Together we will find a cure

My book all about my experience and journey with a brain tumour is now available! All proceeds are going towards Brain Tumour Research.

Available to purchase from Amazon or through myself.

I am also doing a book signing at Woodseats Library on the 16th February 1pm-3pm. Everyone is welcome to come down, snacks and drinks will be provided and Brain Tumour Research merchandise too! It's a great opportunity to get some money raised for such a great charity! Hope to see you there!

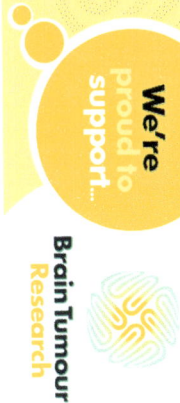

Susan Jones

We're proud to support...
Brain Tumour Research

Together we will find a cure

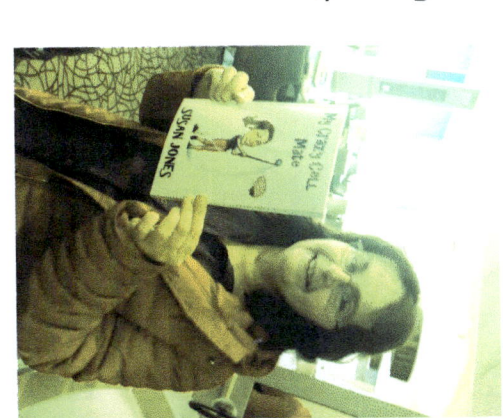

Printed in Poland
by Amazon Fulfillment
Poland Sp. z o.o., Wrocław